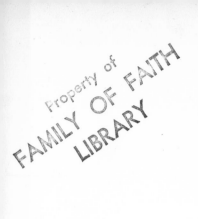

What to Eat and Why

By the Same Author
Earth in Motion

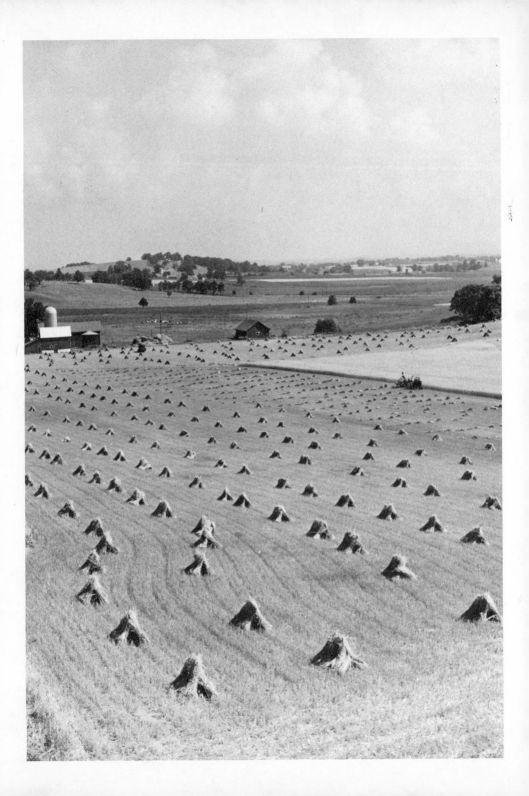

What to Eat and Why

The Science of Nutrition

by R. V. Fodor

illustrated with photographs

William Morrow and Company   New York 1979

Library of Congress Cataloging in Publication Data

Fodor, R. V. What to eat and why.
Summary: Discusses the relationship of basic nutrients to disease
and body disorders. Also outlines the components of a nourishing
diet.
1. Nutrition—Juvenile literature. [1. Nutrition. 2. Diet] I. Title.
TX355.F532   641.1   78-24086
ISBN 0-688-22189-0   ISBN 0-688-32189-5 lib. bdg.

Printed in the United States of America.
First Edition
1 2 3 4 5 6 7 8 9 10

Frontispiece courtesy of United States Department of Agriculture.

For Germaine and John,
two good eaters.

Contents

1
The Science
of Nutrition

Imagine living one hundred years ago. Your life would be greatly different from what it is today. With no automobiles or airplanes, your transportation would be much more limited. You would wear different-style clothes, have far fewer books from which to choose, and you could not enjoy radio or television.

But there is a more important difference. Today, you are likely to grow to be a taller and heavier adult. The records of scientists over the years show that present-day American children grow larger than those who lived before them: young people are up to three centimeters taller and from five to ten kilograms heavier than those of the same age a century ago.

Many reasons are offered to explain this increase

in people's size. Among them are improved housing and sanitary conditions, better programs against diseases, and excellent medical care. But a large and important reason for bigger and stronger people is related to food. Nearly all children today have more to eat and are better nourished. Their eating habits are greatly improved, and good nourishment through food allows for maximum body growth, development, and health.

Achieving the most benefit from the food we eat is of such interest and importance that an entire scientific field is devoted only to food. It is the science of nutrition, and it is concerned with the relationships between life and food.

Nutrition developed from the sciences of chemistry, biology, physics, and anatomy, and it is still closely tied to them. It is an important factor in medicine, public health, and dentistry. In addition, it is involved in many other professions: the agriculturalist is challenged to produce the highest quality crops; the anthropologist is concerned about why people eat the way they do; the economist is interested in improving the eating and living conditions

Inoculation against disease is an important reason for today's children growing up stronger and healthier.
(*World Health Organization*)

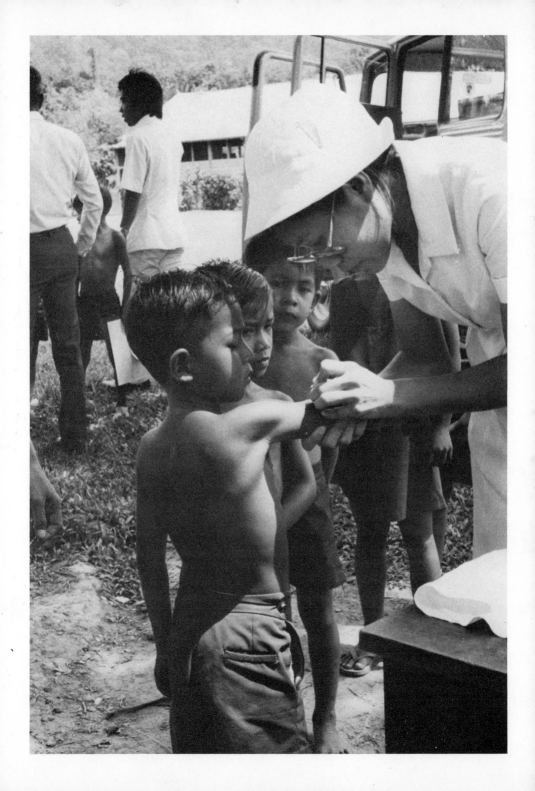

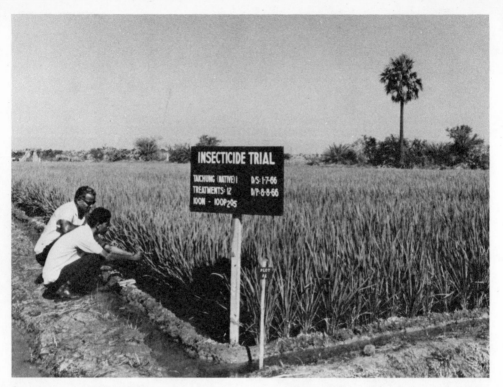

Entomologists, scientists who study insects, experiment with different ways to improve crops and, thereby, nutrition. (*United States Department of Agriculture*)

of entire countries; the demographer works with problems of populations and food supplies. In short, the science of nutrition is important for all human life and for the well-being of everyone.

Although nutrition is a relatively young science, firmly established only in this century, physicians and other scientists have long recognized the importance of diet. Hundreds of years ago it was known that a well-nourished person has good posture, firm muscles, strong bones, and a clear complexion. Lack of energy, frequent illness, and poor posture and complexion were recognized to be signs of a poor diet or undernourishment.

Interest in nutrition was expressed as far back as 2000 years ago. Hippocrates, called the "father of medicine," observed the relationship between the human body and food. He said at that time, "I think of the stomach as a kind of stewpot in which food gets cooked or stewed by body heat," and "Children produce more heat and need more food than adults."

Not until long after Hippocrates, however, did scientific experiments in nutrition begin. One of the most famous early scientists active in such work was Antoine Lavoisier, a Frenchman who lived in the eighteenth century. Though he was a chemist and had performed the experiments that helped develop an understanding of the oxygen content of air, he also had a special interest in nutrition. Lavoisier noted that food eaten was like a fuel in the body and that the more a man worked, the more food he needed. For his contributions to establishing scientific relationships between foods, human lives, and breathing processes, Lavoisier earned the title of the "father of nutrition."

Nutrition as a true science came into being at the turn of the twentieth century. At that time the compositions of certain foods were first determined and the knowledge of particular needs in our diets was acquired. The many vitamins were discovered too. Much of the groundwork was set by people at famous institutions such as Yale and Columbia and by the scientists of the Department of Agriculture. Mary Swartz Rose, who became the first professor of nutrition in the United States in 1921, was an outstanding educator on the subject. In 1918, E. V. McCollum introduced the importance of milk, eggs, and leafy vegetables to help preserve youthful qualities.

Early nutritionists also started to examine the diets of entire communities. For example, some of the work by the first director of research in the United States Department of Agriculture was on the relationships between the health conditions of people in the Appalachian highlands and their food quality. W. O. Atwater noted that poor diet led to the rapid aging of many women's bodies, even though they were young in years. Other early studies demonstrated that the types of foods eaten helped influence how often an individual would suffer from illness. It was also noted that diets around the world varied greatly because of cultural habits and beliefs. For instance, certain societies refuse to eat meat or milk while others exist on bats, mice, or insects.

Nowadays, more than ever, the kinds of food that

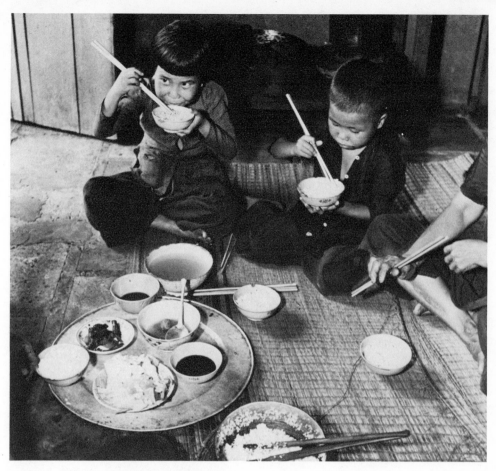

Diets around the world are different. Rice is the basic food in Vietnam. (*World Health Organization*)

we eat are considered the key to proper nutrition and health. Simply eating large amounts of any food is not adequate and is no guarantee of good health. Our well-being depends on eating the necessary amounts of high-quality food.

What determines, then, how nourishing a particular food is? Why do we say that one type of cereal

17

is not as beneficial to our health as another type, or that an apple is a better snack than a candy bar?

The answers lie in the kinds and amounts of nutrients each food contains. Nutrients are the contents of foods that are necessary for the functioning of any living body. They are the materials that nourish our bodies. Nutrients provide the fuel that releases energy for our activities; they are the building material for body upkeep and growth, and they help to control our natural body processes.

We depend on food to supply us with about fifty different nutrients. Fortunately, any one type of food has many nutrients, so we do not have to eat dozens of different types to maintain our health. Milk, for example, contains so many nutrients that it is almost a complete diet in itself. But, in fact, foods vary greatly in their nutritive content and no one food is perfect. We need a variety of food for our well-being.

Scientifically, the nutrients are classified as five major groups: carbohydrates, fats, proteins, minerals, and vitamins. In addition, water is sometimes considered as a sixth major nutrient group. Each of the nutrient groups has a special role in our bodies and is needed to maintain health.

2
The Nutrients

Behind all your activities is energy—the ability to work or play. You can quickly learn about energy by taking a long hike in the mountains or by playing in a fast-moving basketball game. After a certain amount of such rigorous exercise, your body is no longer able to remain active. You simply run out of energy.

With a little rest and perhaps a glass of water, your body may regain some strength. Eventually, however, it will use up too much of the fuel it runs on, and you will not be able to continue your activity. Such a halt happens to people in the same way that it does to cars that use up all their fuel. In the case of human beings, the fuel is food. We supply our bodies with the nutrients in food, and, in turn, we receive energy for action.

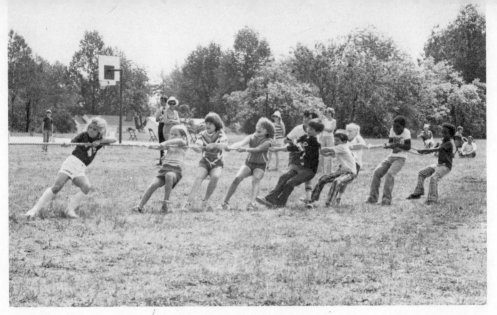

Energy used during a tug-of-war comes from carbohydrates and fats. (*R. V. Fodor*)

The energy may not even be used for exercise. Much of what we produce is used for quiet activities. For example, energy from food is need for making new tissue, for breathing, and for blood circulation. Energy is used while we read and sleep. For these reasons, our bodies require a steady supply of energy-rich foods.

Most of the energy we burn has its origin in two nutrients—carbohydrates and fats. How much energy is provided by each nutrient can be measured in kilocalories, a special unit established by physicists for measuring heat. One kilocalorie is equal to the amount of heat necessary to raise the temperature of one kilogram of water one degree centigrade. Determining the heat the carbohydrates and fats can produce is appropriate to nutrition because heat is given off as our bodies use food.

Each day most young people and adults burn over 2000 kilocalories. We must eat a substantial amount of carbohydrates and fats to supply that kind of energy. Most carbohydrates in our diets come from

A Kenyan farmer stands by his crop of hybrid corn, an important source of carbohydrates.
(*United States Department of Agriculture*)

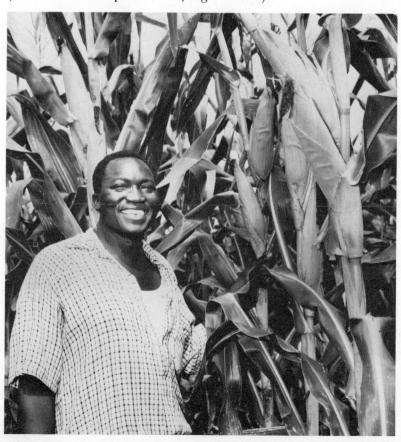

plants such as wheat, corn, potatoes, rice, and fruits. Because these carbohydrate-rich plants grow easily, provide the most food-energy per acre of farmland, and are good tasting, they have been the mainstay of diets across the world since early civilization. In the Orient, for example, rice has been a major part of the diet for thousands of years. Corn was grown in the Americas long before Columbus's visit in 1492. Today we look at carbohydrates as an inexpensive source of energy. Each gram of carbohydrate provides four kilocalories.

The carbohydrate nutrients in foods are composed of three chemical elements: carbon, hydrogen, and oxygen. On the kitchen table the carbohydrate chemical compounds can be recognized as the sugars, starches, and cellulose that we eat.

TYPES OF CARBOHYDRATES

Name	Where found
Fructose	Fruits, vegetables, honey
Glucose	Fruits, vegetables, plant juices
Lactose	Milk, milk products
Galactose	Milk, milk products
Maltose	Grains, malted milk
Sucrose	Ordinary sugar
Starch	Grains, fruits, vegetables, roots
Glycogen	Human liver and muscles (stored for energy)
Cellulose	Grains, nuts, fruits, vegetables

Fructose and glucose are the sugars of fruits and vegetables, which give these foods such appeal to our tastes. Fructose is the sweeter of the two and is also found in the nectar of flowers and in honey and molasses. When eaten, glucose becomes the most important sugar in our bodies. In the bloodstream, it serves as a steady source of energy for body tissues.

Milk products contain sugars, too, known as "lactose" and "galactose," and grains such as wheat have maltose sugar. There is even a similar-sounding scientific name for the ordinary sugar found in the household sugar bowl. It is called "sucrose," and it comes from either sugarcane or sugar beets and can be white or brown in color.

Starch is the most widely eaten carbohydrate. Its main sources are the cereal grains—wheat, corn, and rice—and beans, peas, and edible plant roots.

Cellulose is one carbohydrate we eat regularly, but it provides no energy. Human beings are not equipped to digest this substance. It has, however, a useful role in our diets as bulk or roughage, and it helps keep our digestive systems in good working order. This nutrient is common in fruits, vegetables, cereals, and nuts.

A more concentrated source of food-energy than carbohydrates comes in the form of fats. This nutrient is loaded with nine kilocalories of energy per gram, which is over twice the amount supplied by carbohydrates.

Scientists sometimes use the name *lipids* for this nutrient. The name *fat* is unfortunate because it implies something unfavorable to most people—over-

Rye is a significant source of carbohydrates. (*United States Department of Agriculture*)

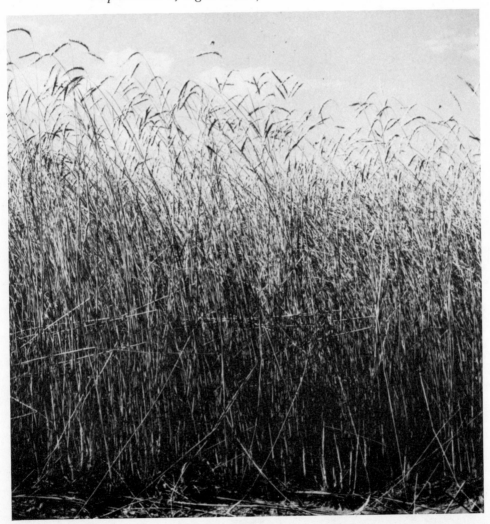

weight. So foods containing fats sound like foods to stay away from.

But eaten in proper amounts, fats serve our bodies well. They are needed not only as fuel for energy, but also serve as the main source of stored, or reserve, energy in our bodies. The storage areas are located under the skin as adipose tissue. There the fat protects us from the changes in outside temperatures and helps us maintain a steady body temperature. Fat also forms the padding on our palms and feet and protectively lines many of our delicate organs, such as the kidneys.

Like carbohydrates, this energy nutrient is chemically made of carbon, hydrogen, and oxygen atoms, and it comes from some vegetables, such as corn. But a good part of the fat we eat is supplied by animals.

Accordingly, nutritionists classify the fats into two groups: vegetable and animal. In either form, fat is a greasy or oily substance that cannot be dissolved in water. Vegetable oil and the white portions of bacon are good examples of vegetable and animal fats that we eat. Other sources of vegetable fats are peanuts and peanut butter, seeds, and nuts; additional animal fats are found in beef, poultry, fish, eggs, and milk products.

The next major group of nutrients is made up of

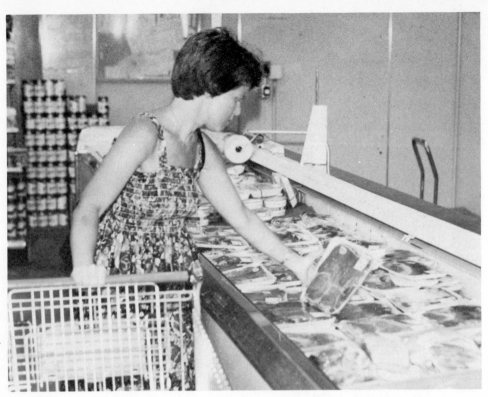

Certain cuts of meat contain a lot of animal fat. (*R. V. Fodor*)

the proteins. Athletes who need muscle development, strength, and stamina for success depend on a combination of hard training and abundant protein. For example, many professional football players recognize that rigorous calisthenics, lifting and pressing heavy barbells, jumping rope, and jogging are only half the battle. Those activities will give them the physical conditioning needed for upcoming games only if they follow up their workouts by eating the proper amount of protein to build and repair body tissue.

Protein, like carbohydrates and fats, is composed of the elements carbon, hydrogen, and oxygen. In addition, it has the element nitrogen, which sets it apart from other nutrients. This chemical difference makes protein the chief building block of our bodies, repairing worn-down tissue, especially the muscles, and constructing new material for growth.

This nutrient is the second most abundant component of our bodies, water being the most plentiful. It composes over one-half of our bodies' dry

Weight lifters rely on protein for developing strength.
(*R. V. Fodor*)

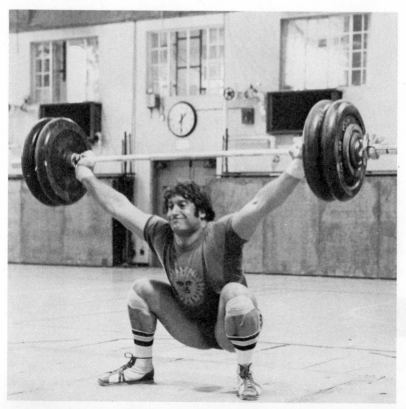

weight, and a sizable portion of it is located in our muscles and bones. In addition, protein is part of many body fluids, such as blood. There it is hemoglobin, the protein that transports oxygen from lungs to tissues and on return trips carries carbon dioxide from tissues to lungs. Protein also serves in the blood as antibodies, or defenders against disease, and it composes parts of many body organs.

The list of roles played by protein in our bodies goes on and on. But if any one is to be singled out and emphasized, it is that of protein in our cells, the microscopic structural units that make up all tissue. In the cells, protein duties vary, depending on the tissue type. In muscles, protein allows the cells to contract and hold water, which gives muscles firmness; the protein in hair, skin, and nail cells forms a hard, protective coating; in blood vessels, protein provides an elastic quality.

Proteins are building blocks. Every day of our lives, this nutrient is needed to maintain and construct tissue. Because of this ability to make body tissue, the greatest amount of protein is needed during the growing years, between birth and the age twenty.

Protein is yet more complex. This nutrient is composed of even smaller structures, or chemical building stones, called "amino acids." In all, scientists have discovered twenty-two amino acids, of which eight are absolutely essential for growth and maintenance.

THE NAMES OF THE ESSENTIAL AMINO ACIDS

Valine
Lysine
Threonine
Leucine
Isoleucine
Tryptophan
Phenylalanine
Methionine

How many of the essential amino acids are present in a protein is the basis for further classification. Protein that contains all eight is called a "complete protein." This kind has high biologic value and is able to maintain life and promote growth. Protein that does not have all the essential amino acids is incomplete; it is not capable of maintaining life or supporting growth.

A variety of foods contain protein, but not too many have it in adequate amounts or in high enough quality for our needs. Almost any animal product, including the dairy products (cheese, cottage cheese, yogurt), is an excellent source and contains complete proteins. On the other hand, proteins in grains,

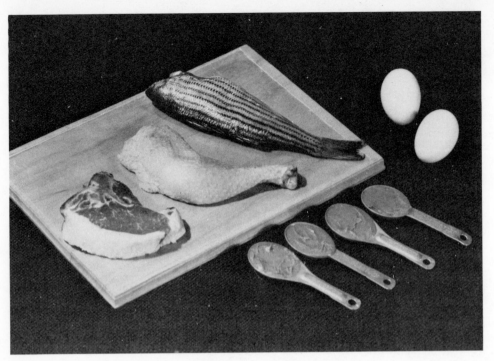

Different forms of protein—meat, fish, eggs, peanut butter.
(*United States Department of Agriculture*)

nuts, and vegetables (with the exception of soybeans) are normally not as high in quality. Foods such as oats, wheat, corn, rye, rice, peanuts, green beans, and peas commonly lack one or more of the essential amino acids. Also, the amount of protein in 100 grams of vegetable or grain is lower than in 100 grams of meat or milk products.

Grain, nut, and vegetable proteins can still be beneficial, however. When two or more of these incomplete proteins are consumed at once, they may combine to form a complete protein. That is, they supplement each other so that our bodies can fully use all amino acids in that food combination. Similarly, when one complete and one incomplete protein are eaten, such as cereal with milk, they may assist each other. The cereal alone may not provide complete protein, but with the milk it can contribute much to a diet.

The soybean is the one vegetable that has protein with quality equal to that of animal protein. In addition, 100 grams of soybeans contain more complete protein than 100 grams of meat. Curiously, this outstanding legume has been overlooked as an important protein source in the Western world, although it has long been popular in the Orient. The United States produces far more than half of the world's soybean crop yet uses it primarily as food for livestock.

Minerals form the fourth major nutrient group. Their importance in our bodies can be demonstrated by a simple experiment that involves tying a bone into a knot. All you need to do is soak a chicken wishbone in a jar of vinegar. About a week later, you can remove the bone, and it will be soft enough to form a knot.

Bones, as well as teeth, use the mineral calcium to make them hard and tough and to assist them in growth. When a bone is put in vinegar, the calcium dissolves out and a once-hard material becomes rub-

31

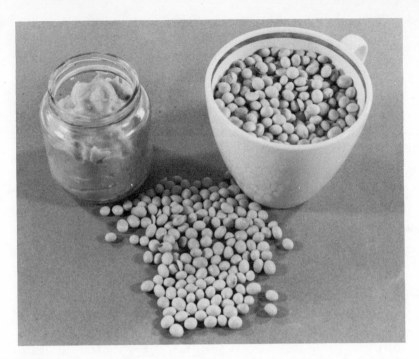

Protein-rich soybeans can be prepared as nutritious baby food. (*R. V. Fodor*)

bery. Clearly we would have no skeletons without calcium.

Calcium is only one of many different minerals needed for good health and growth. As a group, the minerals we acquire from food have two main purposes. One is to make up a large portion of our hard and soft body parts. In addition to the bones and teeth, there are many tissues, such as muscles and glands, that require minerals. Body fluids, such as blood and stomach acid, demand minerals for their makeup too. All told, a fifty-kilogram person carries around about two kilograms of minerals.

In their second role, minerals are needed for certain body functions. For example, our nerves react only with proper amounts of sodium and potassium in the nerve cells. Similarly, most body cells depend on minerals for their operation. The muscle cells contract only with adequate calcium present. This dependence is especially true of the heart, our most important muscle. Minerals are even necessary for turning carbohydrates and fats into energy.

Our bodies are known to need seven minerals in relatively large amounts. They are calcium, phosphorous, magnesium, potassium, sodium, chlorine, and sulfur. Members of this group are called "macrominerals."

Minerals that are necessary in lesser amounts are the microminerals, or trace minerals. This group includes iron, copper, iodine, manganese, zinc, chromium, and fluorine.

The most abundant mineral in our bodies is calcium. It is so plentiful in bones and teeth that many adults have over one kilogram in their body. Calcium is most important to young people, for their bones and teeth are growing rapidly. But adults, too, require a steady supply of calcium. Even though their bones may have stopped growing, there is a continual body process that replaces old bone material with new.

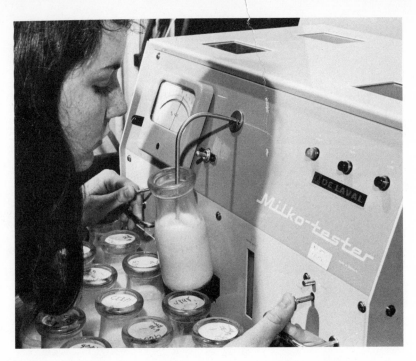

This scientist is testing milk, the best source of calcium, for its fat content. (*United States Department of Agriculture*)

It is easy to include calcium in our diets because the richest food sources are milk and milk products. In fact, no other food offers as much calcium as milk. Next best in supplying this mineral are some of the green leafy vegetables, such as broccoli, and certain fish, such as sardines and salmon.

A diet lacking in calcium can lead to bone and dental problems. An example is periodontal disease. With steady losses of calcium to bones in the jaw, the teeth loosen and the gums become infected.

Yet calcium alone is not enough to make rigid bones and teeth. Phosphorous is required too, for the calcium to combine with. This mineral is the second most abundant in our bodies, found in quantities of about one-half that of calcium.

Phosphorous is also needed for some special body activities. For example, it participates in chemical reactions with carbohydrates and fats to make energy. In addition, there are a number of vitamins that can be of value to us only if they combine with phosphorous in our bodies.

Fortunately, enough common foods contain this mineral so that there is usually no difficulty in obtaining a phosphorous-rich diet. The richest sources are the high-protein foods. Meats and whole-grain cereals have high amounts, as do nuts, peanut butter, eggs, and dairy products.

Iron is another important mineral, and there may be periods when you grow so rapidly that you cannot keep up with your body's demand for it. At such times you could experience an illness known as iron deficiency, or anemia, which causes a general tiredness. To prove the existence of anemia, a physician must determine the amount of hemoglobin present in the blood. There are several foods that can easily cure or prevent this disease. Among them are meats, liver in particular, egg yolks, green leafy vegetables, and dried fruits.

Too little iodine in the diet can present a special

medical problem called "goiter." This ailment is the swelling of the thyroid gland, which is located in the neck. One of the purposes of the thyroid gland is to control growth in children, and it requires sufficient iodine to operate correctly.

In the past, goiter was a worldwide problem, especially in mountainous regions such as the Alps and the Himalayas. Even today goiter is found in certain geographic areas, such as parts of South America, where iodine is rare in the water and soil. Fortunately, it is no longer so much of a problem in the United States. The reason is that iodine is purposely added to table salt. This iodized salt, as it is called, easily provides the iodine necessary for the thyroid gland. The best food source of iodine is seafood.

The history of vitamins, the fifth major nutrient group, began more than 200 years ago with the appearance of two mysterious diseases. During the 1700's, more than half the men on British shipping expeditions would sometimes die of scurvy by the time an ocean was crossed. At the same time, on the other side of the world, Japanese sailors were being struck down by beriberi, an ailment that caused their muscles to break down and anemia to develop.

Entire Latin American villages suffer from goiter due to the lack of iodine in their diets. (*World Health Organization*)

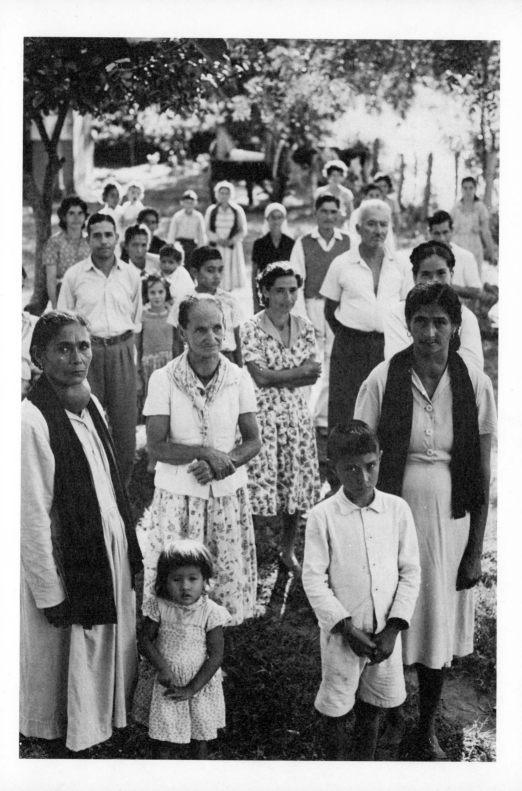

For the longest time scientists were baffled by scurvy and beriberi. Their experience had shown that diseases were caused by bacteria, which did not seem to be true of these two illnesses. Then they learned that scurvy patients were cured when given lemons and oranges to eat, and that people with beriberi recovered when taken off their strict rice diets. Finally, the remarkable discovery was made that these diseases were caused by deficiencies in diet. Certain nutrients—later to be called vitamins—were missing. That breakthrough was revolutionary in the science of medicine.

Vitamins are compounds in foods that are required for our growth, for the utilization of other nutrients, and for the prevention of disease. With one member of the vitamin group missing from a diet, illnesses like scurvy and beriberi can develop.

There are about a dozen important vitamins that we should eat every day, and each one has its special function in our body. Like other nutrients, we obtain most vitamins from animal and plant sources. But each vitamin is needed in only very small amounts, usually much less than one gram per day.

Without these almost microscopic amounts of vitamins in your daily diet, however, your body cannot operate properly. Your eyes, for example, depend greatly on vitamin A for proper vision, and

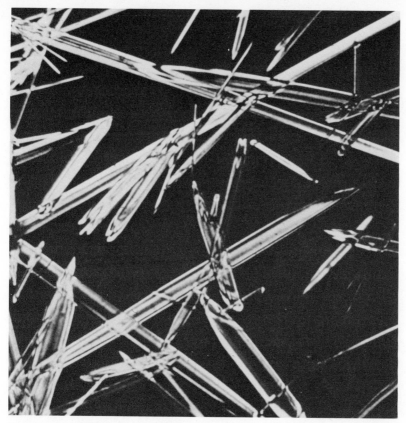

Under the microscope, vitamins appear as tiny crystals. This is Vitamin D_3. (*Hoffman-LaRoche, Inc.*)

your skin would dry up and harden without it. Good food sources of this nutrient are milk, eggs, and liver. Carrots, too, are a major supplier, because they contain a form of vitamin A known as "carotene."

Vitamin K, found in green leafy vegetables, is responsible for the way your blood clots after a cut.

Vitamin D is the only nutrient that can be received simply from sunlight. Its presence in our body is essential to make full use of the calcium we eat. It was not discovered until the early 1900's when a scientist made a surprising observation that cases of the childhood bone disease called "rickets" were rare in regions where sunlight was abundant but common where the sun seldom shone. This information eventually helped determine that rickets was due to the lack of a nutrient identified as vitamin D.

There are eight vitamins we eat that are classified under the B group, better known as the vitamin-B complex. Some members of the complex are referred to by names while others are labeled by the letter B and a number, such as B_{12}.

Thiamin is the vitamin of the B complex known as the "anti-beriberi nutrient," but it is necessary for our utilization of carbohydrates as well. Pork products, cereal grains, and beans are among the best thiamin sources.

We obtain most of vitamin B_2, riboflavin, from milk and liver. Our cell growth depends heavily on this nutrient.

Niacin, found in liver, poultry, and peanut butter, is needed to help use glucose for energy. The importance of niacin in preventing pellagra, a skin disease, was discovered with the help of prisoners. Pellagra was rampant in the South in 1915 when J. Goldberger asked a group of volunteer convicts in a Mississippi jail to eat only special foods as an

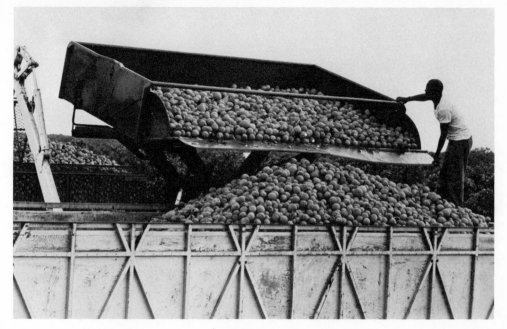

Vitamin C is plentiful in citrus fruit such as oranges.
(*United States Department of Agriculture*)

experiment. Six months later Goldberger was able
to determine that the absence from their diets of
part of the B complex, niacin, was showing up as
pellagra among the prisoners. Thus, pellagra was
proved to be still another nutrient-deficient disease.

The name ascorbic acid is given to the contro-
versial vitamin C. There is no question about the
need for ascorbic acid for cell functions and to prevent scurvy, but there is uncertainty about this
vitamin's role in the battle against the common
cold. Some scientists, such as Nobel laureate Linus
Pauling, argue strongly that vitamin C is helpful
in preventing and curing colds; other researchers

41

claim that there is no scientific proof of this theory. In any case, it is an essential vitamin. A common source for it is in citrus fruits like oranges and grapefruits.

The last nutrient that your body must have large quantities of at all times is water. After all, water makes up far more than half of your body weight, and it has a surprising number of chores to perform each day.

Water is used as building material in every cell. Thus, it is in some body parts that you may never have thought of as containing liquid. Small parts of your teeth, for example, and sizable portions of your bones are made of water. Also, about half of the adipose tissue beneath your skin is water. Even larger amounts of water compose your red blood cells and certain muscles.

The importance of water in your diet begins the moment you eat. The water in your mouth, saliva, quickly acts to soften food, making swallowing easier. Once the food is in your stomach, the water there begins to assist in the digestive process. In fact, water aids the passage of food through your entire body.

During digestion, water (mainly as blood) carries food to cells and, in exchange, takes waste products away. On top of helping transport nutrients and food throughout your body, water itself provides valuable minerals to your diet. Much of what you receive from it depends on where your drinking water comes from, but it is likely to be a major source of at least some minerals, such as fluorine and iodine.

Water also behaves as a thermostat by controlling body temperatures. When you get too warm, water comes out of your skin. This process is known as perspiring, or sweating, and it helps to cool you off. You may perspire several liters of water on hot days or during times when you are very active.

Although you may drink several glasses of water each day, your body is actually getting much more because many foods and drinks supply you with this nutrient. Milk, for example, is almost all water. Soup and watermelon are large sources. Even some of the common garden vegetables, such as cucumber, lettuce, and celery, are composed largely of water.

In the course of identifying the major nutrient groups, scientists learned a number of illnesses are caused by the lack of a specific nutrient. The study of the connection between diet and health has continued, and today many other kinds of diseases are also known to be closely tied to nutrition.

3
Common
Childhood Diseases

Throughout history, all people—kings, queens, and famous presidents alike—have had trouble with their teeth. It seems dental problems go back in time as far as the Egyptian pharaohs. In fact, X rays of mummies have shown that they had cavities in their teeth. One of the best-known facts about George Washington is that he had no teeth of his own, but wore false wooden ones.

Today most people have the greatest number of ailments centered around their teeth. The National Institute of Dental Research reported that, on the average, five-year-old children have three decayed teeth and most teen-agers have more than ten. The reasons for all of these dental problems are greatly related to diets and eating habits.

There are two major types of dental ailments. The

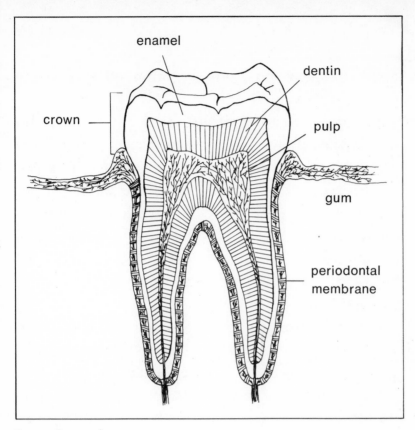

Parts of a tooth.

first is the decay of teeth, or the formation of caries. Because teeth are hard and tough, it may seem that they cannot be damaged, but that is not the case at all. When we eat, the bacteria in our mouth feed on carbohydrates and produce an acid. This bacteria-carbohydrate relationship occurs most readily in the tiny spaces and corners between and on our teeth—the places that are well hidden and difficult to clean and brush. Once this acid forms, which could be as soon as four minutes after eating, it slowly attacks teeth from the outer enamel to the interior pulp.

The type of carbohydrate eaten has much to do with how easily tooth decay can take place. Sucrose, ordinary sugar, is by far the worst for teeth. Thus, candies, most sweet pastries, and the sugar-rich gums, beverages, and cereals are the greatest enemies of our teeth. Starch, on the other hand, is the carbohydrate least harmful to teeth. Most important, though, is not to allow *any* carbohydrate to stick to your teeth after eating.

The second major dental problem lies with tooth settings, the supporting structures that dentists call "periodontal tissue." They are the jaw and the gums.

The periodontal tissues behave just like the bone and soft tissue elsewhere in our body. They require proper nourishment to help build strong teeth and to hold them tightly in place. Periodontal tissues respond to poor nutrition and can become infected and diseased. The result may be loosened teeth that require extraction.

In turn, injured tooth structures can affect our diets. That is, if teeth cause discomfort during eating, some of the most nutritious foods may not be eaten in an effort to avoid pain.

A diet for good teeth and periodontal tissue is most important for young people, whose tooth and jaw structures are growing. It must contain ample amounts of the vitamins A, C, and D, proteins, and the minerals calcium, phosphorous, and fluorine. All of these nutrients contribute to solid tooth, gum, and jawbone development. The necessary foods to eat each day are three to four cups of milk, fruits, green leafy and yellow vegetables, and an egg. Fluorine has been found to be so important in fighting tooth decay that many communities add small amounts to the drinking-water supply just for this purpose.

Even with a diet rich in necessary nutrients, proper brushing and dental care are needed. The American Dental Association recommends brushing your teeth or at least rinsing your mouth with water after every meal. Also, you should visit a dentist every six months for teeth cleaning and inspection.

As important as it is to eat all the nutrients each day, we sometimes have too much of a good thing. There may be days, for example, when we eat more carbohydrates than are really needed. If done only occasionally, there is no harm. But when too many carbohydrates or fats are eaten regularly, problems develop. That is, overnutrition leads to obesity, a body condition in which large amounts of fat have accumulated beneath the skin as adipose tissue.

In science, the Law of Conservation of Energy

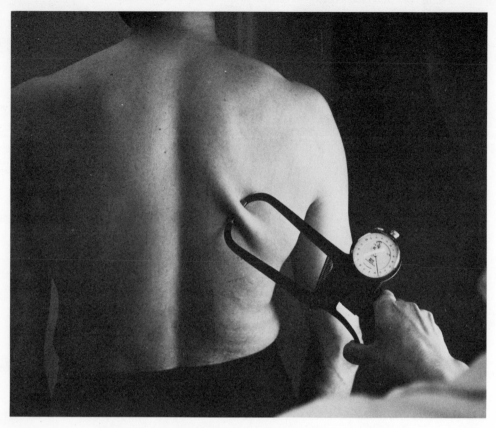

Testing for the thickness of adipose tissue.
(*World Health Organization*)

states that energy cannot be created or destroyed. When applied to nutrition, this law means that if the energy value of the food eaten is greater than the energy a person uses, the remainder will be stored as fat for later use. If the fat is never used and more and more is stored, the food-energy builds up as adipose tissue and obesity results.

Why do people eat more food than they actually need? Are some really more hungry than others?

Many of the reasons for overeating lie in behavior: people often eat even though they are not hungry. Eating can offer comfort when feelings are hurt or during times of frustration or boredom. Someone who lacks affection or recognition at home may turn to food as a substitute for the missing attention. In some cases, a child may become obese because his or her parents use food to express their feelings or as a reward for good behavior.

Sometimes people overeat out of habit. A person accustomed to a bedtime snack may eat one whether the hunger is there or not. The easy availability of food contributes to this problem.

Another major cause of obesity is too little exercise. You must have enough physical activity each day to use up the energy acquired through eating.

Obesity can be cured by controlling the number of kilocalories eaten. More energy must be burned up each day than is eaten, but doing so is not always easy. Preventing obesity is simpler than curing it, and this prevention is especially important during the early years. Evidence indicates that children who are fat often become obese adults. The reasons are partly because obese children develop excessive fat cells that remain with them for life, and partly because children usually carry poor eating habits with them into adulthood.

The health hazards of obesity are many. Excessive body weight can lead to the increased chance of developing diseases such as diabetes and to problems related to the heart, lungs, and blood. There is also great psychological suffering, because obese people are usually not happy about their appearance. In general, very fat people are more prone to accidents and have shorter life-spans.

Curing obesity involves a combination of eating less and exercising more. First, a doctor should be consulted for individual guidance. It is important to cut back on the foods rich in fats and sugars when trying to lose weight. What is eaten, however, should still be good tasting and nourishing, only the amounts should be less.

You should know what the kilocalorie values of foods are. In that way, a record can be kept of how much energy is eaten compared to how much is needed each day for a certain body weight. The fewer kilocalories eaten, the better. As a rule of thumb, remember that about 100 grams of adipose tissue are made for every 800 unused kilocalories. Similarly, by burning up 800 more calories than eaten, 100 grams of body fat will be lost. However, the loss of weight should be gradual. About half to one kilogram of weight loss per week is plenty.

Eating too little can also present a danger. If less

food-energy is taken in than used over a long period of time, an underweight problem may develop. It then could lead to malnutrition, a condition in which one or more of the essential nutrients are missing from the diet. Malnutrition may be marked by

This Indonesian child suffering from malnutrition has a harder time resisting childhood diseases.
(*World Health Organization*)

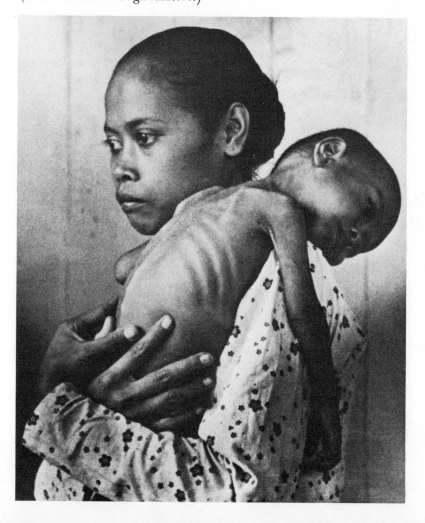

something as simple as anemia, due to not enough iron being eaten, or by a problem as serious as blindness, due to the absence of vitamin A. In any case, the undernourished person is weak and tired, underweight, and frequently ill.

The long-term effects of malnutrition can be especially damaging. Lack of a nutrient in the diets of children frequently shows up later in their adult life. Not enough protein, for example, can lead to poor tooth, bone, and muscle development. In general, they may not grow fully. Malnutrition increases the chances of catching major diseases, too, such as tuberculosis and rheumatic fever. It also makes recovery from any sickness difficult. Even mental development is hurt by undernutrition. Intelligence tests, for instance, have shown that malnourished children score more poorly than healthy children.

There are many reasons for the occurrence of malnutrition. Skipping meals or eating more snacks than meals are major causes. Sometimes ignoring a certain food group, such as the meats, can lead to undernourishment. But the largest reason lies in the food supply: people in many regions of the world do not have enough to eat.

The World Health Organization considers malnutrition to be the number one health problem on the globe. About half of the world's population is

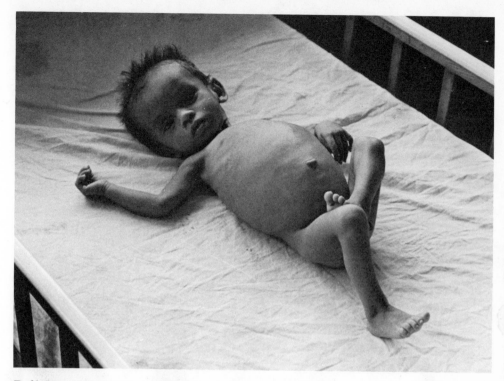

Bolivian child with severe malnutrition caused by intestinal parasites. (*UNICEF*)

undernourished and more than 1000 people die each week as a result. Most commonly, the trouble is protein-calorie malnutrition (p-cm), the lack of adequate protein and calorie intake.

Some diseases that result from eating too little protein are kwashiorkor and marasmus. Both are found mainly among children of age one to six years and are recognized by lack of growth, muscle wasting, unusual swelling, and changes in hair and skin color. In some areas of the world, half the children fail to reach their fifth birthday because of p-cm.

Fortunately, there are cures for malnutrition. Generally, the solution is to begin eating whatever nutrients are missing from the diet. But even though the undernourishment is overcome, permanent damage may have been done. As in the case of obesity, preventing malnutrition is easier than curing it.

Scientists are working to help avoid malnutrition. One example of their progress is an agricultural invention. By crossing wheat and rye grains, a hybrid called "triticale" (pronounced trit-uh-kay-lee) was produced that contains up to twice as much protein as wheat or rye alone. It is a relatively recent development and is not yet widely grown, but the plans for triticale are ambitious. Besides being a new, good-tasting grain, it will help fight the battle against poor nutrition in many undeveloped areas of the world.

Even with new foods like triticale and low-cost protein-rich soybeans, fighting malnutrition is almost like fighting a losing battle. The reason is that the supply of food, although increasing, cannot keep up with the increasing number of people. On the average, two babies are born each second of every day. Unless the rate of population growth lowers, malnutrition is here to stay as a major worldwide health problem.

One of the strangest forms of malnutrition is

anorexia nervosa, a psychiatric disorder in which an individual purposely does not eat, even with ample food at hand. Anorexia nervosa is starvation by choice and is related to severe emotional problems that begin early in childhood.

Most victims of this undernourishment are girls who have difficult family lives as children. When young adults, they develop fears about adulthood, and in trying to live with these fears they acquire peculiar attitudes toward food. Most important on the mind of an anorexia-nervosa victim is to become thin, very thin. One researcher viewed the problem as "starving amid plenty."

The cure for anorexia nervosa is a long process that requires special counseling. Professional help is truly important because many victims of the illness actually starve themselves to death.

4
Body Disorders

There is no question that the way we feel, act, and look is closely tied to our diets. The relationship between health and diet shows up in many ways, and one of the most dramatic is revealed by heart problems. Sometimes they lead to heart attacks and death.

Blood pumped by the heart is the major transport vehicle of our body. Not only does it carry oxygen throughout; it brings nutrients to each cell. Evidence of that nutrient transportation remains along the many kilometers of arteries that the blood travels.

Microscopic examinations of blood vessels have shown that their insides can become coated with fatty deposits called "plaques." The main component of plaque is called "cholesterol," which has its source in the animal fats we eat. After nearly a lifetime of this cholesterol build-up, an artery begins to behave like a dirt-clogged garden hose, and if the blood cannot pass through it, a heart attack results.

Even before a heart attack occurs, plaque in arteries creates a disease called "atherosclerosis." During its slow development over twenty to forty years, atherosclerosis creates many troubles. Blood clots form and interfere with flow, blood pressure increases, and the walls of arteries weaken.

Because of the long development time for this disease, it is mainly found among older adults. Surprisingly, however, the disease begins early in life.

Microscopic view of plaque inside an artery. (*American Heart Association*)

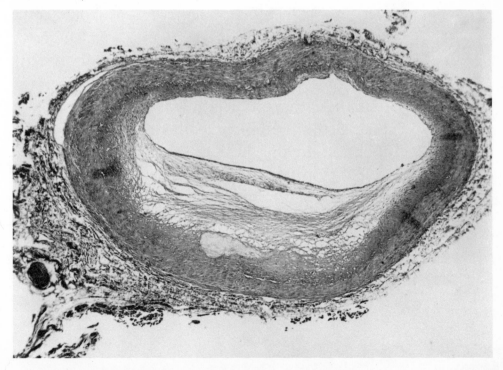

Physicians have noted that fats can start to line artery walls in children only two years old.

Certain populations of the world seem to have fewer cases of atherosclerosis and fewer heart attacks than others. Accordingly, scientists have come to believe that the main causes of this coronary-artery disease are eating and living habits. In particular, a diet rich in fats and a life-style of little exercise are thought responsible.

For these reasons, physicians suggest eating more vegetable than animal fat. Most fat of animal source is chemically saturated, or has an abundance of hydrogen atoms. Scientists have observed that saturated fats, like those from beef and bacon, contain the cholesterol. Therefore, the fats you eat should come largely from vegetable products, nuts, fish, and poultry. Each of these foods contain chemically unsaturated fats and little or no cholesterol.

Another heart problem related to clogged arteries is called "hypertension," or high blood pressure. Sodium in the diet has been singled out as a major cause of this condition. Studies have shown that too much sodium creates high tension and nervousness. Such conditions, physicians warn, bring unnecessary stress to the heart and cause high blood pressure. It is wise, then, to limit the amounts of the sodium-rich table salt you use as seasoning.

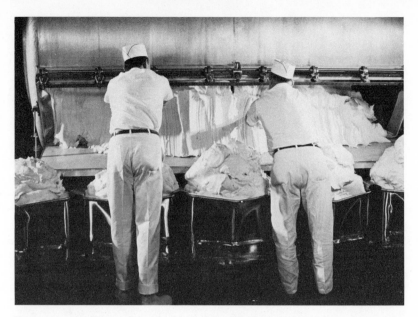

Butter contains ample cholesterol. (*United States Department of Agriculture*)

Yet heredity seems to be closely tied with some heart diseases also. For example, some people will never suffer coronary-artery disease, no matter how much cholesterol they eat. In contrast, other families have a long history of heart trouble. To be on the safe side, nutritionists recommend eating no more than 300 milligrams of cholesterol daily and avoiding much salt. Because exercise appears to reduce fatty deposits in arteries, be sure to remain active.

There is also a close relationship between diet, exercise, and heredity for another common disease known as "diabetes mellitus." This illness is usually called "sugar diabetes." In the case of young people, diabetes is unquestionably hereditary, but diet has much to do with how well a child lives with and controls the problem. Among people over forty years old, poor diet is the chief reason for the outbreak of diabetes.

Bicycling is important exercise for these young diabetics at a camp in Germany. (*World Health Organization*)

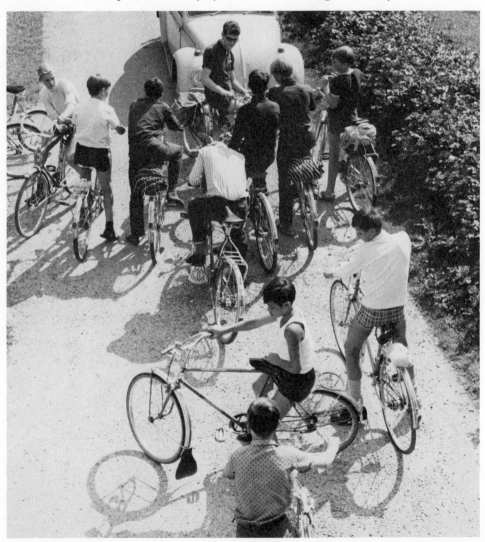

No matter what the age, diabetes is a problem involving an individual's blood sugar. Normally, the glucose that enters the bloodstream from foods eaten is controlled by insulin, a protein produced in the pancreas. Enough insulin is made available to help remove excess glucose from the blood and place it in tissue cells for storage. When too little insulin is produced, or if the insulin is prevented from doing its work, sugar in the blood greatly increases (this condition, whatever its cause, is called "hyperglycemia"). Eventually thirst, fatigue, and weight loss occur. If untreated, diabetes mellitus can lead to atherosclerosis, blindness, and death.

Diabetes is not curable, but it can be controlled. Nearly sixty years ago medical scientists discovered that insulin could be prepared in chemical laboratories and given to diabetics. Taken daily, the insulin keeps the blood sugar of a patient at normal amounts. Yet even with medication, diet plays a great role in the life of a diabetic. Each patient is on a special diet prescribed by his doctor—nourishing but low in fat and carbohydrate.

Good eating habits are an important way to avoid diabetes in later years. The main rule is to limit the amount of food eaten, especially sugar- and fat-rich foods, which readily add to body weight. Obesity is related to diabetes as can often be seen among older people. When some are overweight, mild diabetes occurs; with a loss of body weight, the problem diminishes.

Next to watching your diet, plenty of exercise is important. Not only does physical activity help prevent obesity; it reduces the level of blood sugar.

Exercise is also useful for reducing stress and worry. These problems are frequently found among

A heart patient is tested for breathing, pulse rate, and heart function after exercise. (*World Health Organization*)

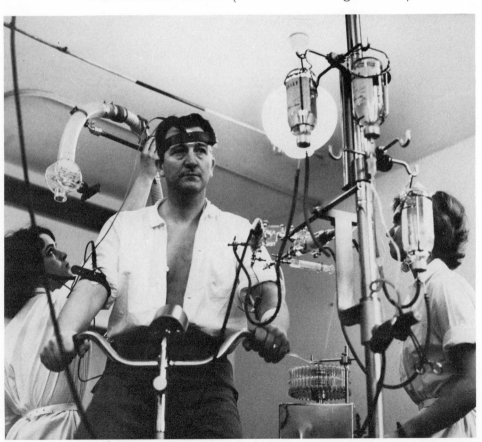

people highly dedicated to their careers, such as hard-working businessmen. The results of these mental pressures can be the development of ulcers—sores inside the stomach.

For this condition, too, diet is important. Foods like fruits, raw vegetables, and carbonated beverages only make ulcers worse. On the other hand, dairy products, particularly milk, help to sooth and heal the stomach sores.

Yet many dairy products can create other medical problems. If more calcium is taken in than can be used, calcium-rich stones may form in the kidneys. Clearly, patients who suffer from kidney stones need to control the amount of calcium in their diet.

Much of your health depends on hereditary traits and on recognizing what diet is best for you. In general, everyone needs certain quantities of the six basic nutrients, but each of us must determine when there is too much or too little of one nutrient or food in our diet. The relationship between nutrition and body disorders is a close one that must be carefully watched throughout life.

5
The Marketplace

A man started drinking a quart of milk each day to satisfy his vitamin-B requirement. He was a late riser because of his job, but the first thing he did every morning was to bring in his bottle of milk from the back porch where it was delivered. He knew the quart of milk contained one and a half milligrams of riboflavin, enough to meet his daily need.

The man was deeply shocked, therefore, when he was told, after years of drinking a quart of milk each day, that he had a nutrient deficiency. There was not enough riboflavin in his diet. "Impossible," he declared. "I drink enough milk to meet the daily need of an adult easily."

With some study of vitamins, the man discovered the reason for his deficiency. Riboflavin is destroyed by exposure to light. The man's milk had stood in sunlight on the porch several hours before he put it in the refrigerator. By then most of the riboflavin was lost.

Many foods lose some nutrient value by the time they are eaten. Some of the greatest losses occur in the home during meal preparations. Cooking heat, for example, destroys amino acids and members of the B complex in meat, and boiling vegetables too long can rob them of their vitamin C.

But even before you bring food into your home, there are plenty of chances for nutrient loss or damage. Long transport times from farm to market can be harmful to vitamins. Being stacked too long on the back of a grocery-store shelf is a sure way to cause spoilage. Even vegetables in a store's cooler begin to wilt in time. Fortunately, many of these problems are avoided by special methods for preserving food.

Heat preservation is used for nearly ten billion cans of food a year in the United States. In this process a can of fruit, for example, is heated and then sealed. In this way the fruit is protected from spoilage by air or bacteria. Home canners use this method, too, because it is inexpensive, efficient, and safe. Actually, it is safe only to a point. There is one serious problem that may develop during the heat preservation of foods: if done improperly, a deadly illness called "botulism" may result.

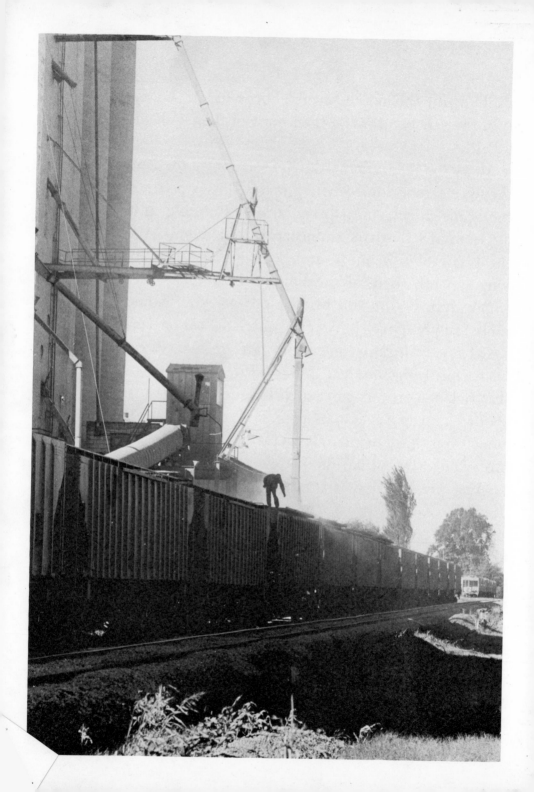

The oldest means of preserving food is drying. By simply placing seeds, grains, and fruits into sunlight, you can remove most of their water content and spoilage is prevented for a long time. A special drying process called "dehydration" removes all the water from food products without changing color or flavor. Foods such as sliced beef, spaghetti, and corn can be dehydrated and eaten months later by adding water to them. Powdered milk is a good example of a dehydrated food found in many homes.

Plain freezing, as you do in your home freezer, is the easiest way to preserve food. The nutritive values of foods are not changed by freezing for the most part. When thawed, however, spoilage can occur quickly, so the food should be eaten soon after.

Certain products require special treatment before freezing. For instance, vegetables must be steamed beforehand so colors and flavors are not changed, despite some loss of vitamin C and minerals. In general, freezing offers the important advantages of long preservation time and convenience. Practically every food and juice can remain frozen and retain most of its nutrients for over a year.

At one time or another, all of us have had in our

The transportation of food over long distances means special care must be taken to prevent spoilage.
(*United States Department of Agriculture*)

homes products labeled "enriched," or "fortified." A package of white flour or a carton of milk carries these words. Do these labels mean that the foods have been changed since their formation? Have the foods been improved as a result? The answers are "Yes" and "Not always." Many products have additives, substances added to change original nutritive values, tastes, textures, or storage life. Some additives are good; some are not.

The need for enriching foods became clear in the 1930's when pellagra was still a common disease in the United States. The cause of this deficiency disease was related to the bread people ate. Although wheat flour is one of the best sources of niacin, this nutrient was not as plentiful in the popular white bread as it could have been. Manufacturers had depleted the original wheat grains of niacin and about twenty other nutrients during preparation of the flour.

Nutritionists realized that controlling pellagra called for the addition of the B complex to wheat flour. In other words, vitamin B_2, niacin, had to be put back. After 1941, nearly all white bread sold in stores was enriched in niacin, and shortly afterward, the number of pellagra cases dropped sharply. Nowadays laws require the vitamin enrichment of all commonly eaten foods, such as white bread, cornmeal, and rice.

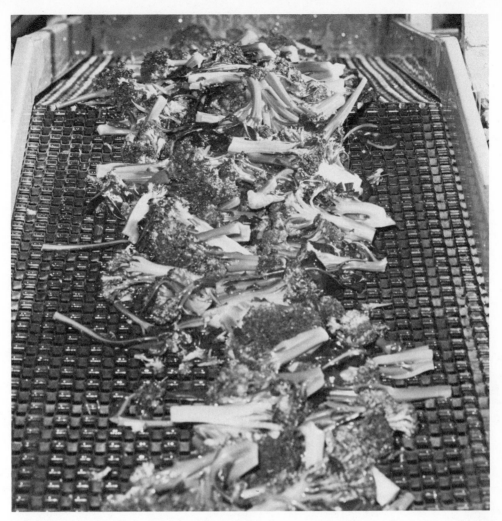

Broccoli is steamed to preserve color and flavor before freezing. (*United States Department of Agriculture*)

Breakfast cereals are not only enriched but fortified. This term means that nutrients never present in the grains have been added. They include iron and calcium and B-complex vitamins.

You can learn for yourself what nutrients are in

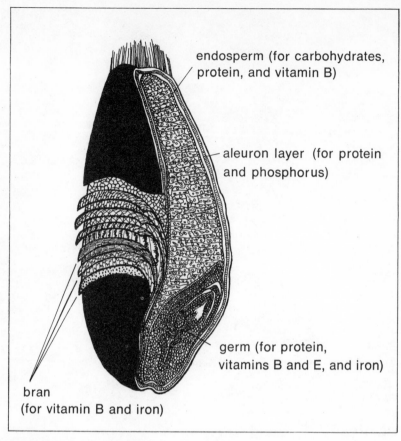

endosperm (for carbohydrates, protein, and vitamin B)

aleuron layer (for protein and phosphorus)

germ (for protein, vitamins B and E, and iron)

bran
(for vitamin B and iron)

Parts of a kernel of wheat.

any breakfast cereal by reading the information on the package. These labels list the ingredients, too, with the most abundant one first on the list. Beware of products that have sugar as the main component. It is true that fortified cereals do contribute to the vitamins needed in your daily diet, but many offer large amounts of sugar and very little protein.

One may wonder why whole grains of wheat are processed to remove the nutrients, especially if the flour made from the wheat is later to be enriched. The reason is preservation: removing the germ of the wheat gives flour a longer life on the shelf.

But there are serious faults with this processing system. For example, food manufacturers cannot put the protein back in, nor do they add back all of the B complex purposely removed.

You should know whether grain products such as flours and breakfast cereals were made from whole grains or from refined grains. Whole grains are those in which all original nutrient content is present. Refined grains have lost much of their original nutrients during processing by food manufacturers. Clearly, whole grains are preferred as nutrient sources. For preservation, keep whole-grain products refrigerated.

Any kind of food spoils if left too long in the cupboard or refrigerator. To preserve foods of all types, a variety of chemicals are added to them. These additives have names like nitrates, sulfites, benzoates, and they help keep foods free of mold and from becoming rancid. All of them have been approved for use as preservatives in the United States.

Additives are used for more than enriching, fortifying, and preserving. Nearly 2000 different ones are put in our foods for the sole purpose of making them taste or look better. Sweeteners such as sugar and corn syrup are most widely used, with salt in second place. These two additives are so common that the average American eats about ten kilograms of sugar and six kilograms of salt as additives each year.

Other additives include the carbon dioxide that makes soda bubble and yeast dough rise. Most of the rest are chemicals such as acids, bases, and neutralizing agents. They affect the flavor, texture, and

Sugar cane is the source of the most common food additive. (*United States Department of Agriculture*)

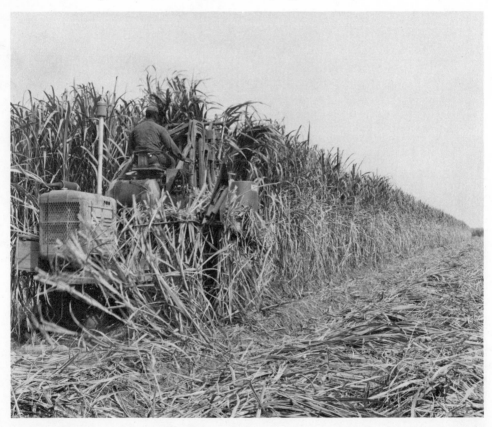

color of the food we eat and are not put in food for health purposes. They only give the products more appeal to our eyes and our taste.

The Food and Drug Administration controls what additives and how much of each can be used. Quantity is certainly important because too much of almost any additive can be harmful. To ensure the safety of additives in any amounts, the FDA has asked scientists to check each one by experiments. As a result, several changes have been made in the Government's original list of approved additives. Some were found to bring possible harm. Cyclamates, for example, had to be outlawed. These artificial sweeteners were in wide use before they were shown to cause cancer in animals.

Research chemist analyzes a low-calorie dessert topping for additives. (*United States Department of Agriculture*)

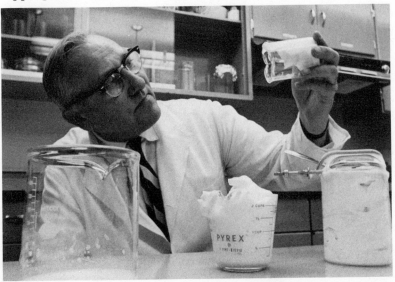

Further criticism was brought against food additives by Dr. B. F. Feingold in connection with a widespread health problem. In the early 1970's, he suggested that additives are responsible for hyperactivity (hyperkinesis), an illness that may affect several million children. A hyperactive child is usually unable to concentrate, sit still for long periods, or sleep well. The child also is clumsy and readily gets angry. But the connection between this illness and food additives remains open to question. The latest scientific studies have failed to show a relationship between diet and hyperactivity.

The foods we eat come from many different parts of the country and sometimes from outside the United States. Long transportation times and long display times make preservative additives necessary. Although some people would rather not have anything added to their foods, many additives are beneficial. Because of them, foods now are much safer from invasion by bacteria than they were a generation ago. Those that enrich and fortify food contribute to our health. Sweeteners and color additives, however, have little to do with good nutrition.

6
Selecting
a Nourishing Diet

At school age, you are one of the most active people in the world. A major portion of your life is probably spent running, climbing, learning new games and sports, and participating in athletic programs. In addition, the school years are the time of greatest body growth and development. Your muscle size and strength are greatly increasing, your body composition and shape are changing, and your are growing new teeth and bones. For all these reasons, a nutritious diet is very important for you. Eating well during the early years will help set the foundation for a healthy, active adult life.

Nutritionists say that an adequate diet is composed of all the necessary nutrients in the proper amounts. In practical terms, you should eat servings from four food groups each day: milk, meat, vegetable-fruit, and cereal. These categories allow a wide choice of foods.

Making the four-group plan the framework of your daily diet may be easy enough, but how are you to know how much of each food type to eat? Should you drink as much milk (for minerals) as your parents, or eat as much meat (for protein) as an older brother? One way to answer these questions is to refer to the special lists of Recommended Dietary Allowances provided by the Food and Nutrition Board of the National Research Council.

As the RDA listings point out, age and size make a difference in how much of the different nutrients we should eat. For example, seven- to ten-year-old children need 800 milligrams of calcium to stay in good health, while eleven-to-fourteen-year-olds need 1200 milligrams.

But you don't have to live each day by lists and numbers. Just remember to eat at least one serving from each food group daily. In that way, you will most likely avoid a diet deficiency.

Besides eating the proper amounts of nutrients, you should develop good eating habits. You should eat three solid meals a day and perhaps a few nutritious snacks. Distributing the nutrients over the day rather than eating most of them at only one or two meals is important for keeping your body sup-

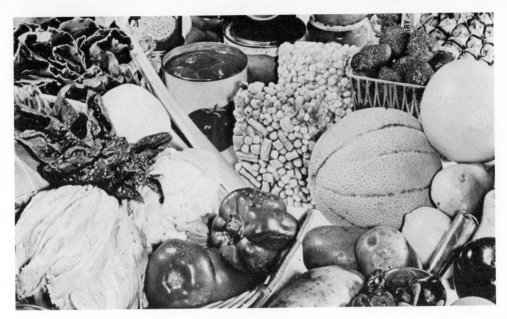

Vegetables and fruits—one of the four food groups.
(*United States Department of Agriculture*)

plied with a steady flow of nourishment. In addition, you should not miss any meals.

Begin each day with a wholesome breakfast. Eat fruit or drink a glass of fruit or vegetable juice. Suggested fruits are grapefruit, cantaloupe, oranges, peaches, and pears. For juice, consider grapefruit, orange, pineapple, or tomato. Equally nourishing choices to eat are a bowl of a whole-grain cereal, toast, biscuits, or muffins made from whole-grain flour, one or two eggs, or a meat like bacon or ham. Drink one cup of milk, either with cereal or alone. It could be whole milk, low-fat whole milk, skim milk, powdered milk, or buttermilk; all are equally nourishing.

The breakfast cereal granola is simple to make in your kitchen. You can purchase the ingredients from a health-food store.

GRANOLA

3 cups rolled oats
2 cups wheat flakes
(rye or triticale flakes may be substituted for oats or wheat)
⅓ cup sunflower seeds
¼ cup sesame seeds
⅓ cup wheat germ (or bran)
¾ cup vegetable oil
½ cup honey

Combine the oats, wheat, seeds, and wheat germ in a mixing bowl, and stir them together. Pour vegetable oil over the combination, and mix it in thoroughly. Add the honey and mix well. Spread out the granola mixture on a cookie sheet with sides. Bake at 325 degrees until lightly toasted, about twenty to thirty minutes. Before serving as a cereal, you can add raisins.

A nourishing lunch at school or at home might consist of one or two sandwiches made with whole-grain bread. The sandwich filling should have protein—a meat product, including fish and poultry, cheese, or peanut butter. Alternatively, substitute one cup of yogurt for a sandwich. Eat vegetables, such as raw carrots or celery, or a bowl of green beans or peas. A fruit—like an apple, orange, pear, or peach

—served with cottage cheese is good. Dessert could consist of a cookie or two, pudding, nuts, or a moderate serving of ice cream. Drink one to two cups of milk.

The evening meal, or main meal whenever it is eaten, should be balanced with meat, vegetables, and dairy products. Hearty dinners could include a serving of beef, pork, ham, chicken, turkey, or fish as the main course. For side dishes, choose among potatoes (preferably not French fries), sweet potatoes, corn, rice, macaroni, turnips, or stuffing. Green vegetables can be eaten as salad or as a side dish.

All four food groups are likely to be part of a nourishing school lunch. (*R. V. Fodor*)

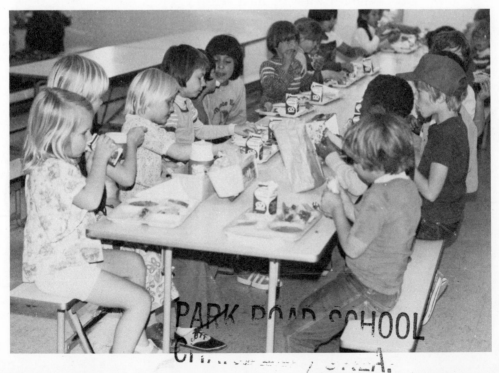

Green beans, peas, broccoli, or spinach are good choices. A nourishing dessert could be pudding, pie, cake, cottage cheese or yogurt mixed with fruit. Drink one to two glasses of milk.

Light eating after school or before bedtime can be an important part of a good diet, as long as the snack is wholesome and does not contribute to an overweight problem. Raw vegetables, fruits, and nuts are among the best snack foods. Yogurt and cheese are healthful, too. You can prepare some nourishing snacks yourself.

celery sticks stuffed with peanut butter or cream cheese

dried fruits (raisins, dates, apricots)
   mixed with a puffed cereal

mixed nuts, seeds, and raisins

apple slices coated with peanut butter and raisins

popcorn

whole-wheat crackers and cheese

fresh fruit in yogurt or cottage cheese

NO-BAKE PEANUT BUTTER LOGS

1 cup powdered milk
¼ cup honey
1 cup peanut butter
2 tablespoons wheat germ, toasted
½ cup sesame seeds

Mix together all ingredients except sesame seeds. Shape the mixture into tiny logs and roll in sesame seeds. Refrigerate the logs before eating.

HIGH-PROTEIN COOKIES

1 cup shortening
1 cup brown sugar
2 eggs
1 teaspoon vanilla
2 cups whole-wheat flour
1 teaspoon baking powder
½ teaspoon baking soda
¼ cup wheat germ
½ cup sunflower or sesame seeds
1 cup quick-cooking oats
¾ cup milk
1 cup raisins

Cream the shortening and sugar in a mixing bowl. Add eggs and vanilla and mix well. Sift together the flour, powder, and soda; add this blend and other ingredients to the first mixture and mix all ingredients well. Drop a teaspoon at a time onto a greased cookie sheet. Bake at 375 degrees for ten to twelve minutes.

Sometimes certain life-styles influence diets. Athletes, for instance, need to eat larger amounts of certain nutrients. Where strength is important, as in football or wrestling, the diet should emphasize high-quality protein foods such as meat, fish, eggs, and milk. In general, one gram of complete protein

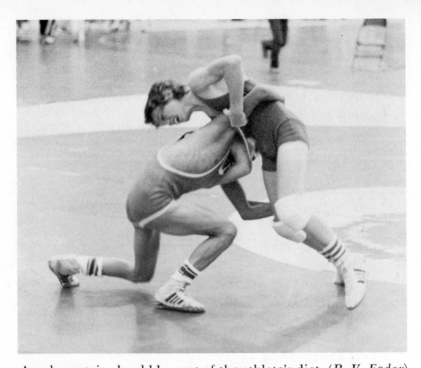

Ample protein should be part of the athlete's diet. (*R. V. Fodor*)

should be eaten for every kilogram of body weight. That is, if you weigh forty kilograms, eat about forty grams of protein daily.

For the kind of stamina required for basketball, track, and soccer, add to your food intake of nourishing carbohydrates and fats. They will help to obtain extra kilocalories and energy. Good sources are fruits, dairy products, nuts, and peanut butter.

What about the pregame meal? What should it consist of? Food before sports activity should be the type that is easily digested. Generally, food that is high in protein leaves the stomach more quickly than food that is rich in fat. A combination of protein and fat takes the longest to digest. Note that you should eat more than three hours before your game.

Meat is one part of the four-group plan that some people do not eat for religious or cultural reasons. This custom does not prevent them from attaining a nourishing diet, however, as long as other protein sources make up for the absence of meat. Dairy products, for example, are good meat substitutes. Many strict vegetarians eat ample supplies of soybeans and combinations of legumes and grains for their protein needs.

In recent years several specialized diets have become popular, and more are sure to come. These fads largely intend to help a person lose weight or avoid additives. Often a fad diet suggests eating an abundance of one nutrient at the expense of another. Some diets encourage eating super amounts of protein and almost no carbohydrates. Others stress no fats or food grown in soil free of fertilizers.

Common sense must be used in these cases. The need for the proper amounts of the necessary nutrients is basic. If a diet is truly nourishing, it contains the balance of nutrients that our body demands. When weight loss is desired, eat fewer kilocalories and exercise more, but make sure to include all important nutrients in your diet.

One rule holds for all diets, however: Avoid foods that have almost nothing to contribute to your being. Popular names for these foods are "empty calories," "junk foods," and "foodless foods." These names are appropriate. Table sugar is a good example, for it has absolutely no nourishing contents—no vitamins, no minerals, no protein—only plenty of calories in the form of carbohydrate. Thus, the calories in sugar are empty.'

Certainly we need carbohydrate in our diet. But you should choose a food that contains minerals or vitamins or protein as well. The calories you eat should come from foods that have nourishment.

There are plenty of products that have earned the title of empty calories or junk food. A number of them, such as soda pop, potato chips, candy, doughnuts, and sweet rolls, are the favorites of a great many young people. In fact, junk foods appeal to the sweet taste of almost everyone, for nearly all of them contain sugar.

At present, there is much discussion and concern over sugar and the dangers that lie among its empty calories. The greatest criticism of it charges that it is the main cause of obesity. Sugar provides too many calories too easily.

Sugar can also lead to malnutrition, because eating empty calories can readily meet daily kilocalorie requirements. For young people unaware of nutrition, satisfying a sweet tooth frequently comes before eating hearty meals. Sugar is responsible for many dental problems too. More recently, some doctors have linked sugar intake with heart diseases.

Many people add another empty-calorie product to their diet. This one, alcohol, can present very serious health problems.

Alcohol is a major ingredient in beverages such as beer, wine, and whiskey—all products that some people drink frequently and in large quantities. There are several reasons people drink alcoholic beverages —to be sociable, to relax or ease emotional distress, or to satisfy taste and thirst.

In any case, some people do not know how to limit the alcohol they drink. They make it a major part of their daily diet and drink enough to meet their daily energy needs. Alcohol contains seven kilocalories per gram. If a person drinks too much of it, not enough protein, vitamins, and minerals will be included in the diet, and malnutrition results.

Protein deficiency is usually the biggest concern with alcoholism. The combination of alcohol plus the absence of protein damages the liver in particular. Cirrhosis is the disease that results. It destroys the liver by replacing the cells with scar tissue and commonly brings death.

Other medical problems occur with alcoholism. They include hypertension, severe vitamin deficiency, and the loss of memory that marks the first step toward brain damage.

Alcoholism is a dangerous disease. Treating the medical problems that develop is possible, but there is a special difficulty to overcome: drinking alcohol becomes a habit. A person can come to desire alcohol as strongly as water. Clearly, then, the most important step in curing alcoholism and regaining health is learning to break the drinking habit.

The path to good health begins with proper nutrition. You should eat and drink adequate amounts of carbohydrates, fats, proteins, minerals, vitamins, and water every day. You also should not overeat any special food types; otherwise more kilocalories are consumed than can be burned off or one nutrient becomes neglected.

But good health does not stop with food. Eating the necessary nutrients must be combined with proper dental habits, exercise each day, and a sound sleep every night. Together they provide the keys to an active life that will help one avoid illness.

CARBOHYDRATE CONTENTS IN 100 GRAMS OF CERTAIN FOODS

Food	Carbohydrate in grams
Sugar	99.5
Candy (butterscotch)	94.8
Honey	82.3
Crackers (graham)	73.3
Crackers (saltine)	71.5
Jams	70.0
Cake (angel food)	60.2
Candy (sweet chocolate)	57.0
Bread (white)	50.4
Potato chips	50.0
Cake (pound)	47.0
Pie (apple)	38.1
Potatoes (French fried)	36.0
Pizza (cheese)	28.3
Rice (white, cooked)	24.0
Bananas	22.2
Potato (baked)	21.1
Ice cream	20.8
Peanuts (raw)	18.6
Walnuts	14.8
Apple	14.5
Soybeans (cooked)	10.1
Soda pop (cola) (3½ ounces)	10.0
Beets (red)	9.9
Green beans (raw)	7.1
Liver (beef)	5.3
Milk (whole) (3½ ounces)	4.9
Yogurt	4.9
Cheese (creamed cottage)	2.9
Cheese (cheddar)	2.1
Egg	0.9
Butter	0.4
Hamburger (cooked)	0.0

KILOCALORIE CONTENTS OF 100 GRAMS OF CERTAIN FOODS

Food	Kilocalories	Food	Kilocalories
Butter	716	Milk (whole) (3½ ounces)	65
Walnuts	628	Apple	58
Peanut butter	581	Yogurt	50
Potato chips	568	Beets (red)	43
Peanuts (raw)	564	Soda pop (cola) (3½ ounces)	39
Candy (sweet chocolate)	528	Green beans	32
Cake (pound)	473		
Crackers (saltine)	433		
Cheese (cheddar)	398		
Candy (butterscotch)	397		
Sugar	385		
Crackers (graham)	384		
Honey	304		
Jam	272		
Cake (angel food)	269		
Bread (white)	269		
Pie (apple)	256		
Pizza (cheese)	236		
Liver (beef)	229		
Hamburger (cooked)	219		
Ice cream	193		
Egg	163		
Rice (white, cooked)	119		
Soybeans (cooked)	118		
Cheese (creamed cottage)	106		
Potato (baked)	93		
Bananas	85		

Food	Fat in grams	Food	Fat in grams
Oil (salad and cooking)	100.0	Cake (angel food)	0.2
Butter	81.0	Bananas	0.2
Margarine	81.0	Green beans	0.2
Mayonnaise	79.9	Beets (red)	0.1
Walnuts	59.3	Milk (skim) (3½ ounces)	0.1
Peanut butter	49.4	Potato (baked)	0.1
Peanuts (raw)	47.5	Sugar	0.0
Potato chips	39.8	Honey	0.0
Candy (sweet chocolate)	35.1		
Bacon (fried)	33.3		
Cheese (cheddar)	32.2		
Cake (pound)	29.0		
Hamburger (cooked)	20.7		
Crackers (saltine)	12.1		
Egg	11.5		
Sardines (dry)	11.1		
Pie (apple)	11.1		
Liver (beef)	10.6		
Ice cream	10.6		
Crackers (graham)	9.4		
Pizza (cheese)	8.3		
Cheese (creamed cottage)	4.2		
Salmon (pink, raw)	3.7		
Milk (whole) (3½ ounces)	3.5		
Yogurt	3.4		
Bread (white)	3.2		
Peas (green)	0.4		

Food	Cholesterol in milligrams
Egg yolk	1500
Egg (whole)	550
Liver (raw)	300
Butter	250
Lobster meat	200
Oyster meat	200
Shrimp	125
Cheese (cheddar)	100
Lard and other animal fat	95
Beef	70
Chicken	60
Ice cream	45
Cheese (creamed cottage)	15
Milk (whole) (3½ ounces)	11
Milk (skim) (3½ ounces)	3
Margarine (vegetable)	0

PROTEIN CONTENTS IN 100 GRAMS OF CERTAIN FOODS

Food	Protein in grams	Food	Protein in grams
Soybeans (raw)	34.1	Soda pop (cola) (3½ ounces)	0.0
Chicken (cooked, no skin)	31.6	Sugar	0.0
Peanut butter	27.8		
Wheat germ	26.6		
Peanuts (raw)	26.0		
Beef (chuck, cooked)	26.0		
Cheese (cheddar)	25.0		
Tunafish (canned)	24.0		
Salmon (canned)	21.7		
Walnuts	20.5		
Sardines (canned)	18.8		
Rolled oats	14.2		
Whole wheat flour	13.3		
Egg	12.9		
Rye	12.1		
Soybeans (cooked)	11.0		
Bread (whole wheat)	10.5		
Wheat flour (refined)	10.5		
Bread (white)	8.7		
Lima beans (cooked)	7.6		
Ice cream	4.0		
Milk (whole) (3½ ounces)	3.5		
Broccoli (cooked)	3.1		
Potato (baked)	2.6		
Rice (white, cooked)	2.0		
Green beans (raw)	1.9		
Lettuce (raw)	1.2		

Index

95